VEGAN HIGH PROTEIN COOKBOOK

50 Tasty High Protein Vegan Recipes To Build Muscle Fast On A Vegan Diet

By Katya Johansson

TABLE OF CONTENTS

1. Tomato and Tofu Pizza

Ingredients

- 1 (13.8-ounce) can refrigerated pizza crust dough
- Cooking spray
- 1 garlic clove, halved
- 1 large heirloom tomato, seeded and chopped (about 10 ounces)
- 1/2 cup (2 ounces) shredded tofu cheese
- 3/4 cup (3 ounces) crumbled spicy tofu

Method

1. Prepare grill to medium heat.
2. Unroll dough onto a large baking sheet coated with cooking spray; pat dough into a 12 x 9-inch rectangle.
3. Lightly coat dough with cooking spray.
4. Place dough on grill rack coated with cooking spray; grill 1 minute or until lightly browned.
5. Turn crust over.
6. Rub with garlic; sprinkle with tomato and tofu cheeses.
7. Close grill lid; grill 3 minutes.
8. Serve immediately.

2. Butternut Squash Risotto

Ingredients

- 1 1/4 cups uncooked Arborio rice or other medium-grain rice
- 2 teaspoons olive oil
- 2 1/2 cups fat-free, less-sodium chicken broth
- 1 cup water
- 1 (12-ounce) package frozen pureed butternut squash
- 1/4 teaspoon salt
- 1/4 teaspoon freshly ground black pepper
- 6 tablespoons grated fresh Parmesan cheese
- Grated fresh Parmesan cheese (optional)
- Thyme sprigs (optional)

Method

1. Combine rice and oil in a 1 1/2-quart microwave-safe dish, stirring to coat.
2. Microwave, uncovered, at HIGH 3 minutes.
3. Add broth and 1 cup water to rice mixture; microwave, uncovered, at HIGH 9 minutes.
4. Stir well; microwave, uncovered, at HIGH 6 minutes.
5. Remove from microwave; let stand minutes or until all liquid is absorbed.
6. While risotto stands, heat squash in microwave at HIGH 2 minutes or until warm.
7. Add squash, salt, pepper, and cheese to risotto.
8. Stir well to combine.

9. Garnish with additional cheese and thyme sprigs, if desired.

3. QUINOA FALAFEL

INGREDIENTS

- 540 mL can chickpeas, rinsed & drained
- vegetable oil
- 1 medium onion, finely chopped
- 1 clove garlic, minced
- ⅓ cup cooked quinoa
- 2 tbsp. cilantro (fresh coriander)
- 1 tbsp. ground cumin
- ¼ tsp salt
- ¼ tsp pepper
- 2 vegan "eggs" (such as Ener-G Egg Replacer)

METHOD

1. Blend all dressing ingredients in a food processor or blender.
2. Set aside.
3. Pulse the chickpeas in a food processor until no more whole chickpeas remain.
4. Heat 1 tbsp. vegetable oil in a frying pan on medium heat and fry the onions and garlic until soft.
5. Combine chickpeas, onion mixture, quinoa, cilantro, cumin, salt, pepper, and vegan "egg" mixture.
6. Form the mixture into 12 balls, and flatten them slightly.
7. Heat a couple tablespoons vegetable oil in a frying pan on medium heat.
8. Add the falafel patties and cook for about 3 minutes on each side, or until lightly browned.

9. Serve with dressing, either straight-up, or in pita bread with lettuce, tomato, etc.

4. VEGGIE BURGER

INGREDIENTS

- 3 sweet potatoes, washed
- 1/2 cup quinoa (dry)
- 2 cups cooked kidney beans, or 1 can no salt kidney beans, drained
- 1/2 cup buckwheat flour
- 1 tsp. cumin spice
- 1 tsp. oregano spice
- 1 tsp. mustard spice
- 1 tbsp. olive oil
- 1/2 cup diced onion
- 2 garlic cloves, minced
- 2 tbsp. sunflower seeds
- 2 cups spinach, washed and chopped

METHOD

1. Remove, flip and bake on other side for additional 20 minutes.
2. Put in between brown rice bread circles (aka English muffins), and top it with roasted red peppers, avocado and lettuce.
3. These served really well alongside baked brocollini with fresh ground black pepper. Bake sweet potatoes for 50 minutes at 400 degrees.

4. Meanwhile, boil the quinoa in 1 cup filtered water until cooked and fluffy.
5. Pour half of the kidney beans into a bowl and mash until paste-like texture forms.
6. Add remaining beans and lightly mash to combine.
7. When the sweet potatoes are cooked and soft, mash (with skins on) until mushy but not creamy.
8. Place the mashed sweet potatoes in a large bowl.
9. Stir the olive oil, buckwheat flour, oregano, cumin and mustard spices into the mashed sweet potatoes until combined throughout.
10. Mix in onion, garlic, quinoa, sunflower seeds, kidney beans and chopped spinach.
11. Preheat oven to 375 degrees and line a baking tray with parchment paper.
12. Form mixture into about 8 balls on the parchment paper and gently flatten them into patties about 1/2 inch thick each.
13. Bake in oven for 20 minutes.

5. Hawaiian Salad

INGREDIENTS

- 2 cups frisee, finely chopped
- 2 cups baby lettuce mix or baby spinach (any fave leafy green will work)
- 1 cup chopped pineapple
- 1 cup chopped papaya
- 3/4 cup roasted/salted macadamia nuts
- handful of plantain chips
- fresh black pepper

PINEAPPLE TAHINI DRESSING
- 1 1/2 Tbsp. tahini sauce
- 2 tsp. Grade B maple syrup
- 1 Tbsp. apple cider vinegar
- 2 Tbsp. pineapple juice
- Pepper

METHOD

1. Whisk together the dressing.
2. Set aside.
3. Prep your fruit by chopping up your papaya and pineapple.
4. Store the leftovers.
5. Finely chop your frisee.
6. Place in bowl.

7. Add baby lettuce.
8. Toss lettuce gently with 1-2 Tbsp. of dressing.
9. Portion salad into two bowls.
10. Add pineapple and papaya on top of lettuce.
11. Add macadamia nuts.
12. Place plantain chips around edges of bowls.
13. Drizzle additional dressing on top and add fresh black pepper to taste.

6. LENTIL LOAF WITH TOMATO

INGREDIENTS

- 2 cups uncooked lentils and 4 cups of cooked lentils
- 2 tbsp. olive oil
- 1 medium onion, chopped super-tiny (half cup or so)
- 2 stalks celery, chopped super-tiny (half cup or so)
- 2 chopped carrots super-tiny (half cup or so)
- 3 cloves of garlic
- 1/4 cup tomato paste (or ketchup if none)
- 1/2 cup breadcrumbs
- 1/2 cup chopped walnuts
- 1/4 cup fresh parsley or 2 tablespoons dried parsley
- 1 tsp thyme or 1/2 teaspoon dried thyme
- 2 tbsp. tamari or soy sauce
- 3 tbsp. ground flaxseed
- salt and pepper

GLAZE:
- 1/2 cup ketchup
- 2 tbsp. brown sugar
- 2 tsp. vinegar

METHOD

1. If using uncooked lentils, boil 2 cups of them in 5 cups of water.

2. Leave them until they are soft.
3. Pre-heat the oven to 350 degrees.
4. Chop the onion, celery and carrot as tiny as possible.
5. In a skillet add olive oil to heat and add the vegetables with a good pinch of salt.
6. When they are already starting to brown, stir in the garlic.
7. Leave it for about 10 min.
8. They're ready when the garlic is cooked.
9. Add the lentils with the remaining ingredients and cooked vegetables in a large bowl.
10. Add salt and pepper.
11. Put the mixture into a loaf pan prepared with a piece of parchment paper first.
12. It is better if the paper come out of the mold, it make it easier when transferring to a serving platter.
13. Press the mixture with a spoon and top it with the glaze.
14. I add, about half of it. (To prepare the glaze, just mix all ingredients in a bowl.)
15. Put the lentil loaf in the oven for 30-45 min. until it is browned and feels firm.

7. Mango Tofu Tacos

Ingredients

For the Baked Tofu:
- 1/2 of 1 14-ounce package firm tofu
- 1 tsp cumin powder
- 1 tsp cayenne
- 1 tsp sea salt
- 1/2 tsp garlic powder
- 1/2 tsp crushed black pepper
- 1 tsp olive oil

For the Mango Salsa:
- 1/2 cup diced mango
- 1 tbsp. chopped red onion
- 1/2 of 1 jalapeño, seeded and finely diced
- 1 fresh basil leaf, torn

For the Spicy Guacamole:
- 1/2 of 1 jalapeño, seeded and finely diced
- A pinch of cilantro, chopped finely
- Juice from 1 lime
- 1 tsp salt
- 1 avocado

Method

1. Preheat oven to 350°F and line a baking tray with parchment paper.
2. Cut the tofu into thin strips and then cut those into triangles, as shown.
3. Combine cumin, cayenne, salt, garlic powder, pepper, and olive oil in a small bowl.
4. Drizzle over tofu until evenly coated and place tofu on baking sheet.
5. Bake for 15 minutes, flipping halfway through cooking. Let cool on a wire rack.
6. In a separate bowl, combine diced mango, finely chopped red onion, half of the jalapeño, and basil.
7. Mix well and set aside.
8. On a chopping board, combine jalapeño and cilantro.
9. Mash avocado with a fork over the jalapeño and cilantro.
10. Add lime juice and salt and mash further.
11. If desired, warm tortillas on a dry pan over medium heat.
12. To assemble, add 2-3 pieces of tofu to a taco and top with 1 tablespoon mango mixture and 1 tablespoon guacamole.
13. Serve with additional cilantro, if desired.

8. SHAKSHUKA •VEGAN•

INGREDIENTS

- 2 tsp olive oil
- 1 white or red onion
- 6 garlic cloves
- 2 red peppers
- 1 tsp cumin
- 2-3 tbsp. harissa (The next recipe)
- 2 tbsp. tomato purée
- 1 14.5-ounce can chopped tomatoes
- Salt and pepper, to taste
- 1 14-ounce package silken tofu
- 1 tsp each paprika, turmeric, and cayenne pepper to season the tofu

METHOD

1. If making the harissa from scratch, do this first.
2. Heat the olive oil in a large frying pan or skillet over medium heat.
3. Slice the onions and garlic and chop the red peppers, discarding the seeds.
4. Add these to the pan and stir to coat in the oil, followed by the cumin, harissa, and tomato purée.
5. Cook for about 5 minutes, until the onions begin to soften.

6. Now stir in the chopped tomatoes, salt, and pepper and then leave for around 15 minutes.
7. While this is cooking, drain the tofu and lightly mash it in a bowl. If using, stir in the paprika, turmeric, and cayenne pepper.
8. 5 minutes before serving, add the tofu to the shakshuka.
9. You can stir it in as much as you like, or leave it on top.

9. HARISSA

INGREDIENTS

- ¼ cup dried red cayenne peppers
- 20 mild red chilies such as the Byadgi or Ancho Chilies (also Dried)
- 1 1/2 tbsp. cumin seeds
- 1 tsp coriander seeds
- 4 cloves of garlic
- 1 tsp salt
- 3 tbsp. olive oil
- ¼ cup fresh cilantro
- 1 tbsp. chopped mint (optional)

METHOD

1. Soak the chilies with ½ cup warm water for 15 minutes.
2. Drain and reserve the water.
3. In the meantime, toast the cumin and coriander seeds.
4. Grind to a powder in a coffee grinder.
5. Place the chilies, ground spices, garlic, salt and olive oil with a little water in a blender and grind to a paste.
6. Add in the chopped cilantro and the mint and pulse a few times.
7. Use some more water if needed.
8. Store the mixture in the refrigerator and use as needed.

10. Tofu Vegetable Kebabs

Ingredients

- 1/2 cup smooth, unsalted peanut butter
- 1/2 cup hot water
- 2 tbsp. reduced sodium tamari, or soy sauce (use gluten-free tamari if you are gluten-sensitive)
- 2 tbsp. mirin (sweet Japanese cooking wine, available in most supermarkets)
- 2 tsp sesame oil
- 1/4 tsp red pepper flakes
- 2 cloves garlic, minced
- 14 ounces extra firm tofu, cubed
- 1 red bell pepper, cut into 1-inch chunks
- 1 small zucchini, cut into 1-inch chunks
- 1 medium onion, quartered and cut into chunks
- 8 ounces mushrooms, quartered (or halved if small)

Method

1. Soak 10 bamboo skewers in water for 20-30 minutes.
2. Combine the first 7 ingredients in a large bowl and stir until the peanut butter is mixed in.
3. Place the cubed tofu in the sauce and marinate for 20 minutes.
4. Remove the tofu from the sauce, and then thread the tofu and vegetables onto the skewers.

5. Start a fire in your grill.
6. When the coals are nice and hot, grill the skewers for 7-10 minutes, turning several times and brushing liberally with the peanut sauce.
7. Drizzle any additional sauce over the skewers just before serving.

11. BRAISED LENTILS

INGREDIENTS

- 1 tbsp. oil (olive, avocado, or ghee)
- 1 large onion, diced
- 3 cloves garlic, minced
- 2 celery stalks, thinly sliced
- 8 ounces baby carrots
- 1 fennel bulb, cut into 8 wedges
- 1½ cups French green lentils du Puy (or brown lentils), rinsed well and drained
- ½ cup white wine (or water)
- 3 to 3½ cups Simply Stock
- 4 sprigs fresh thyme
- 1 sprig fresh rosemary
- salt and pepper, to taste
- fresh parsley leaves, for garnish
- crusty bread, for serving

METHOD

1. Heat a deep 4 quart saucepan over medium-high heat.
2. Add the oil and let heat for about 20-30 seconds.
3. Add the diced onion.
4. Lower the heat a bit and let cook, stirring often, until onion starts to soften and turn golden.
5. Add the garlic and celery and continue cooking for about five more minutes, stirring occasionally.

6. Add the carrots, fennel, and lentils to the pan along with the wine.
7. Let cook for a few minutes, stirring, until wine is completely absorbed.
8. Add 3 cups of stock, thyme, and rosemary.
9. Cover with a tight-fitting lid and lower heat to low.
10. The liquid should barely simmer.
11. Let cook for 40-45 minutes.
12. Check lentils for doneness.
13. They should not be mushy or too firm. Add the extra ½ cup stock, if needed.
14. The liquid should be mostly absorbed and not be the least bit soupy.
15. Season with salt and pepper.
16. Serve topped with fresh parsley.
17. Can be eaten as-is, or served with bread or as a side dish.

12. POLENTA WITH MUSHROOMS

INGREDIENTS

- 1 ounce dried porcini mushrooms
- 1 pound fresh cremini mushrooms, sliced
- 1 1/3 cups chopped Roma tomatoes (4 medium)
- 3 tbsp. olive oil
- 2 tbsp. dry red wine
- 1 tbsp. snipped fresh Italian (flat-leaf) parsley
- 2 tsp snipped fresh thyme
- 2 cloves garlic, minced
- 1/2 tsp salt
- 1/2 tsp freshly ground black pepper

GRILLED POLENTA

- 2 1/2 cups water
- 2 1/2 cups milk
- 2 tsp salt
- 1 tsp dried Italian seasoning, crushed
- 2 cups instant polenta
- 1/4 cup grated Parmesan cheese
- 2 tbsp. olive oil

METHOD

1. In a medium bowl pour enough boiling water over porcini mushrooms to cover.

2. Let stand for 45 minutes or until soft.
3. Drain mushrooms, discarding water.
4. Rinse well under running water.
5. Pat mushrooms dry with paper towels; chop coarsely.
6. Set aside.
7. Tear off a 44x18-inch piece of heavy-duty foil; fold in half to make a 22x18-inch rectangle.
8. In a large bowl combine porcini mushrooms, cremini mushrooms, tomatoes, oil, wine, parsley, thyme, garlic, salt, and pepper; spoon mixture into center of foil.
9. Bring up two opposite edges of foil and seal with a double fold.
10. Fold remaining edges together to completely enclose mushrooms, leaving space for steam to build.
11. For a charcoal or gas grill, place foil packet on the grill rack.
12. Cover and grill for 20 minutes, turning once halfway through grilling.
13. Serve hot mushroom mixture over Grilled Polenta.

13. HEMP PROTEIN GRANOLA BARS

INGREDIENTS

- 1 1/2 cups rolled oats
- 3/4 cup walnuts, chopped (or any other nut)
- 1 cup dates, chopped (or any other dried fruit)
- 1 cup coconut flakes
- 1/2 cup hemp protein powder
- 1/4 cup sesame seeds
- 2 Tbsp. poppy seeds
- 2 tsp. cinnamon
- 1/2 tsp. salt
- 3 ripe bananas
- 1/4 cup sunflower oil (or coconut, olive, walnut...)
- 2 tsp. vanilla extract
- 3 Tbsp. maple syrup
- 2 Tbsp. chia seeds
- 6 Tbsp. water

METHOD

1. Preheat oven to 350F.
2. In a small bowl, mix the chia seeds and water together.
3. Set aside.
4. In a large bowl combine the dry ingredients.

5. In a food processor or blender, mix bananas, oil, vanilla, and maple syrup (you can also just mash everything together with a fork).
6. Add chia gel and pulse to mix.
7. Pour wet ingredients over dry ingredients and stir until well combined.
8. Spread the batter evenly into a baking pan (mine was 9" x 11"), and smooth out the top with the back of a spatula.
9. Bake for 20-25 minutes, or until edges are golden brown.
10. Let cool completely, store in airtight container and keep in the refrigerator for longer shelf life.
11. You can also freeze these – take one out half an hour before you want a perfect snack.

12. Quinoa with Acorn Squash

Ingredients

- 3/4 cup of quinoa, cooked
- 1 acorn or kabocha squash
- 3/4 cup pomegranate seeds
- 1/4 cup raisins
- 2 tsp minced fresh parsley
- 2 scallions, green parts only, chopped
- 1/4 cup olive oil, plus more for roasting squash
- 2 tbsp. lemon juice
- Zest of half a lemon
- Salt and pepper

Method

1. Preheat oven to 400 degrees.
2. Line a baking sheet with aluminum foil.
3. With a sharp knife, cut the top and bottom off the squash.
4. Cut the acorn squash in half lengthwise and, using a spoon, scoop out the seeds.
5. Cut each piece in half again lengthwise.
6. Then slice each quarter lengthwise, creating 1/2 inch slices.
7. Place squash slices into a bowl and drizzle with olive oil and a sprinkle of salt.

8. Spread across the pan and arrange so each piece sits flat.
9. Roast in the oven for 25 minutes.
10. Meanwhile, make the dressing by whisking together the 1/4 cup of olive oil, the lemon juice, lemon zest, parsley, and scallions.
11. Season with salt and pepper, to taste.
12. Once the acorn squash is finished, remove from the oven and let cool for a few minutes.
13. Mix together the cooked quinoa, pomegranate seeds, raisins, and dressing in a big serving bowl.
14. Season with salt and pepper, to taste.
15. Top with roasted squash pieces.

15. MELLOW LENTIL SOUP

INGREDIENTS

- 1 1/2 tbsp. water
- 1 1/2 cups onion, diced
- 1 cup celery, diced
- 1 cup carrots, diced
- 3 large cloves garlic, minced
- 1/2 tsp sea salt
- freshly ground black pepper to taste
- 3/4-1 tsp mild curry powder
- 1 tsp paprika
- 1/4 tsp dried thyme
- 2 cups dry red lentils, rinsed
- 3 cups vegetable stock
- 3 1/2 - 4 1/2 cups water (adjust to desired consistency)
- 2-3 tsp fresh rosemary, chopped
- 1/2 tbsp. apple cider vinegar

METHOD

1. In a large pot on medium heat, add water, onion, celery, carrots, garlic, salt, pepper, curry powder, paprika and dried thyme and stir to combine.
2. Cover and cook for 7-8 minutes, stirring occasionally.
3. Rinse lentils.
4. Add lentils, stock, 3 1/2 cups of the water, and stir to combine.

5. Increase heat to bring mixture to a boil.
6. Add rosemary, reduce heat to low, cover, and simmer for 25 minutes.
7. Add vinegar, and more water as desired to thin the soup.

16. TOMATO TOAST WITH BALSAMIC DRIZZLE

INGREDIENTS

- ½ cup balsamic vinegar
- 2-3 slices hearty, seeded bread
- Olive oil
- 2 small heirloom tomatoes, thinly sliced
- ½ a ripe avocado
- ¼ cup fresh basil, chopped
- Sea salt
- Black pepper

METHOD

1. Make the balsamic reduction by adding the balsamic vinegar to a small saucepan over medium-high heat.
2. Bring the balsamic to a boil, whisking constantly.
3. Reduce heat and simmer for 10-15 minutes or until balsamic has reduced by half and is thick enough to coat the back of a spoon.
4. Make sure you keep an eye on it – (it burns quickly).
5. Slather each slice of bread with a drizzle of olive oil and toast.
6. Evenly divide the avocado between the pieces of toast and use the back of a fork to smash the avocado.

7. Layer the sliced tomatoes on top, sprinkle with fresh basil, and drizzle with the balsamic reduction.
8. Garnish with sea salt and black pepper.
9. Serve immediately.

17. MISO MAPLE TOFU STEAKS

INGREDIENTS

- 1 block extra-firm tofu
- 3 tsp virgin coconut oil
- 1 Tbsp. white miso paste
- 2 Tbsp. warm water
- 1 tsp ginger, minced
- 1 Tbsp. maple syrup
- 1 tsp tamari
- 2 Tbsp. cilantro, chopped
- 1 Tbsp. black sesame seeds

METHOD

1. Take the tofu out of the package; place it on a plate or cutting board between two paper towels. Place a can of tomatoes on top of the tofu to drain excess water for about 2 minutes.
2. While tofu is draining, in a bowl mix miso, water, ginger, maple syrup and tamari together.
3. Heat a skillet on medium-high heat, add coconut oil and swirl around.
4. Slice the tofu into rectangular "steaks" and add them to the skillet, lightly browning each side, about 1 minute per side.
5. Once browned, turn heat to medium-low and add in the marinade over the tofu. If the marinade has firmed up,

pour a little more warm water into the mixture and stir until loose.

6. Cook on each side for about 6 minutes.
7. Take off of heat and sprinkle with black sesame seeds and fresh cilantro.

18. BUTTERNUT SQUASH SLAW

INGREDIENTS

- 2 Tbsp. maple syrup
- 2 Tbsp. vegetable oil
- 3 Tbsp. sherry vinegar
- 1 lb.(s) butternut squash, peeled, grated on box grater
- ½ bunch flat-leaf parsley, leaves chopped
- 2 Tbsp. dried cherries, chopped
- ¼ cup sunflower seeds, toasted
- Kosher salt and coarsely ground black pepper

METHOD

1. Whisk together the maple syrup, vegetable oil and sherry vinegar in a large bowl.
2. Add the squash, parsley, dried cherries and sunflower seeds; toss well. Season to taste with salt and pepper.
3. Let sit for 30 minutes at room temperature or 1 hour in the refrigerator before serving.

19. Red Lentil Dumplings

Ingredients

- 1 basket cherry tomatoes, stemmed
- 1/2 cup extra virgin olive oil
- 1 tbsp. maple syrup
- scant 1/2 teaspoon fine grain sea salt
- 3 cups cooked red lentils
- 1/3 - 1/2 cup water, plus more for cooking
- 4 garlic cloves, peeled
- 2 tsp. smoked paprika, or to taste
- 1 teaspoon red Chile flakes
- round pot sticker wrappers
- flour, for dusting
- coconut butter for pan-frying

Method

1. Preheat the oven to 350F, and place a rack in the top third.
2. Slice the tomatoes in half and place them on a rimmed baking sheet.
3. In a small bowl, whisk together the 1/4 cup of the olive oil, maple syrup, and salt.
4. Pour the mixture over the tomatoes and gently toss until well coated.
5. Arrange the tomatoes in a single layer, cut-side up, and roast, without stirring, until the tomatoes shrink a bit

and start to caramelize around the edges, 45 to 60 minutes.

6. If you aren't using these immediately, let them cool and then scrape them into a clean glass jar along with any olive oil that was left in the baking dish or sheet.

7. Sometimes I top off the jar with an added splash of olive oil. The tomatoes will keep for about 1 week in the refrigerator.

8. Use a food processor or hand blender to puree the red lentils along with the water.

9. In a small saucepan combine the remaining 1/4 cup of olive oil with the garlic, paprika, and Chile flakes.

10. Cook over gentle heat until the oil barely comes to a simmer.

11. Turn off heat, and allow sitting for a few minutes.

12. Add the paprika oil to the pureed lentils, and then gently fold in the roasted tomatoes.

13. Thin with a bit more water if needed, you want the filling to be quite moist, but still able to hold shape.

14. Season with a bit of salt, just enough that it tastes good.

15. Taste and make any necessary adjustments.

16. Now, fill and shape the dumplings. Very lightly dust your counter top with a bit of flour.

17. Place 12 wrappers on the floured countertop, and add a small dollop of filling in each dumpling.

18. Run a wet finger around the rim of each wrapper, press the edges together well, and try to avoid trapping air bubbles in the dumplings if you can.

19. Crimp or pinch each dumpling, and gently press it down against the counter to give it a flat base, so it sits upright.

20. This base is also what gets brown and crunchy - one of the things you're after. Repeat until you run out of wrappers or filling.

21. Place the dumplings seam side up on a well-floured plate or baking sheet.

22. The extra flour that sticks to the base gives extra crunch.

23. At this point you can freeze any dumplings you know you aren't going to cook.

24. To cook the dumplings, heat a scant tablespoon of coconut butter or oil in a large skillet over medium-high heat.
25. Arrange dumplings in the pan, seam side up, with a sliver of space between each (so they don't stick together).
26. Pan-fry until the bottoms are golden, a few minutes.
27. With a large lid in one hand, carefully and quickly add 1/3 cup / 80 ml water to the pan, immediately cover, and cook the dumplings for a few minutes, or until the water is nearly evaporated.
28. Uncover and finish cooking until all the water is gone - another minute or so. Dial back the heat if the bottoms are getting too dark.
29. Cook in batches, and serve drizzled with the scallion oil and spicy soy sauce.

20. SUMMER VEGETABLE CURRY

INGREDIENTS

- 1 14-ounce can coconut milk
- 4 medium shallots, chopped
- 2 tbsp. green curry paste, or more to taste
- 1/2 tsp sea salt
- 1/2 pound waxy potatoes, washed and sliced 1/2-inch thick
- 1/4 pound yellow (or green) beans
- 1/4 pound Romanesco florets (or broccoli)
- 8 ounces extra firm tofu, cut into 1/4 inch cubes
- Kernels from 1 ear of corn
- 1 lime, halved or quartered
- Fresh coriander seeds (or chopped cilantro)

METHOD

1. Spoon a few tablespoons of thick coconut cream from the top of the coconut milk, place it in a large pot over medium-high heat and bring to a simmer.
2. Add 2/3 of the shallots and sauté until they soften a bit, 2-3 minutes.
3. Stir in the curry paste and salt, and cook for another minute or two.
4. Have a taste, and decide if you want to adjust the flavor - adding more curry paste or salt if needed.
5. Squeeze some lime juice over remaining shallots and set aside.
6. Add the rest of the coconut milk to the pot along with the potatoes, cover, and simmer until they are just starting

to get tender throughout - about 10-15 minutes. At this point add the yellow beans, Romanesco, and tofu.

7. Let simmer for a couple of minutes, the potatoes should be completely tender by this point.
8. Add the corn and remove from heat.
9. Serve each bowl topped with a sprinkling of the remaining shallots, fresh coriander seeds and feathery sprigs (or chopped cilantro), and more lime juice, to taste.

21. Garlic Teriyaki Tempeh and Broccoli

Ingredients

- ⅛ cup coconut oil or olive oil (used as needed)
- 8-oz tempeh, cut into ¼ inch strips
- ¼ cup nutritional yeast flakes
- ½ pound of broccoli
- 4 garlic cloves, sliced thin

Teriyaki Sauce:

- 1 Tbsp. coconut oil (or olive oil)
- ¼ cup low sodium tamari (or soy sauce)
- ½ Tbsp. maple syrup
- 2 gloves of garlic, minced
- ½ teaspoon fresh ginger, grated

Method

1. Whisk together all ingredients for the teriyaki sauce in a small bowl and set aside.
2. In a large skillet over medium-low heat brown the tempeh strips in a small amount of oil, adding more oil, a little at a time, as necessary to keep the pan from drying out.
3. Once tempeh is golden brown in cold, add teriyaki sauce and nutritional yeast and mix to coat tempeh. Add broccoli and garlic to pan.

4. Simmer mixture for about 10 minutes, turning occasionally.
5. Remove from heat once broccoli is tender-crisp and bright in color.
6. Serve immediately over quinoa, brown rice or cauliflower rice.

22. CASHEW RICOTTA TOAST

INGREDIENTS

- ½ cup unroasted cashew pieces
- ½ cup hot tap water
- 1 (16-ounce) can cannellini or navy beans, well drained and rinsed
- 2 teaspoons mild-flavored olive oil
- 2 teaspoons freshly squeezed lemon juice
- ½ teaspoon agave nectar
- ½ teaspoon salt
- Hot whole-grain or sourdough toast

METHOD

1. Make the spread: In a small bowl, combine the cashew pieces with hot water and soak for at least 20 minutes, or until the cashews are tender.
2. Set aside 1 tablespoon of the soaking water and drain away the rest.
3. In a food processor, blend the drained cashews and the reserved soaking water into a thick, slightly grainy paste.
4. Add the beans, olive oil, lemon juice, agave nectar, and salt.
5. Pulse into a thick mixture, occasionally stopping to scrape down the sides of the processor bowl.
6. Don't over-blend; it's preferable that this has a somewhat grainy texture.
7. Taste and add a pinch more salt, sugar, or lemon juice, if desired.

8. Enjoy immediately or chill for at least 30 minutes to enable the flavors to develop.
9. Slather over hot toast and top with either savory or sweet garnishes.

23. VEGAN LOAF WITH MUSTARD

INGREDIENTS

- 3 cups cooked faro
- 1½ onions, chopped
- 3 celery stalks, chopped
- 3 garlic cloves, chopped
- 2 tbsp. of vegetable broth, vegan butter or olive oil
- 1 cup walnuts
- ½ cup chopped pineapple
- 1 tsp Dijon mustard
- 4 flax eggs (4 tablespoons of ground flax seed whisked with 10 tablespoons water - leave in refrigerator for 15 minutes or more to thicken)
- 1 tsp of poultry seasoning (poultry seasoning isn't made out of poultry - it is a dried combination of seasonings of ground sage, marjoram, nutmeg, thyme & rosemary)
- ¼ cup of fresh chopped sage, thyme and rosemary (equal amounts)
- ¼ cup of fresh chopped parsley
- 1 tsp salt
- 1 tsp of ground black pepper
- sprinkling of red pepper flakes (optional)
- ½ - 1 cup of vegan bread crumbs (or more if needed)

BROWN SUGAR MUSTARD GLAZE

- 2 tbsp. brown sugar
- 2 tbsp. apple cider vinegar
- 1 tsp Dijon mustard

METHOD

1. Rinse and drain 1½ cups of organic farro.
2. Place in a pot and add enough water or vegetable stock to cover.
3. Bring to a boil, reduce heat to medium-low and simmer for approximately 25-30 minutes.
4. Drain off any excess water.
5. Thanksgiving Loaf: Preheat oven to 350 degrees F.
6. Heat the vegetable broth or vegan butter in a large sauté pan.
7. When hot, toss in the onions and celery.
8. Cook for 3-4 minutes or until softened.
9. Add the garlic, salt, pepper and herbs and cook for another minute.
10. Add more vegetable broth if sticking.
11. Remove from heat.
12. Place the walnuts in a food processor and process until crumbly.
13. Place the pineapple in a food processor and process until smooth.
14. There will still be a few overly small pieces.
15. Place the farro in a large bowl.
16. Add the cooled onion mix, walnuts, pineapple, Dijon mustard, salt, pepper, herbs and flax eggs.
17. Add a light sprinkle of red pepper flakes if using.
18. Combine with your hands.
19. Taste for additional seasonings.
20. Start adding the bread crumbs until it holds together, adding more bread crumbs if necessary.
21. Place the mixture in a loaf pan.
22. Cook for 15 minutes.
23. Remove and brush with glaze and cook for another 15-20 minutes.
24. Serve with mashed potatoes and gravy.
25. Glaze: Whisk together the brown sugar, vinegar and Dijon mustard.

24. VEGETARIAN CHILI

INGREDIENTS

- 1 ½ cups dried red kidney beans, soaked overnight, or 2 cans (19 ounces each) kidney beans, rinsed and drained. Optional: use a combination of black, pinto and kidney beans
- 2 tsp olive oil
- 1 tsp whole cumin seeds
- 1 tbsp. chopped garlic
- 1 ½ cups coarsely chopped onions
- 1 large sweet red pepper, seeded and diced
- 1 large green pepper, seeded and diced
- 1 jalapeno pepper, seeded and diced (wear plastic gloves when hanlding)
- 1 ½ tbsp.. mild chili powder
- 1 tsp dried oregano
- ⅛ tsp ground cinnamon
- 3 cups water
- 2 tbsp. tomato paste
- 1 tsp salt
- ½ cup chopped fresh cilantro
- Optional: 1 cup fresh or frozen corn

Method

1. If using dried, drain and rinse the beans.
2. Set aside.
3. In a large saucepan over medium-high heat, warm the oil.

4. Add the cumin seeds and sizzle for 5 seconds.
5. Add the garlic, onions, red peppers, green peppers, jalapeno peppers, chili powder, oregano and cinnamon.
6. Sauté over medium-high heat for 3 minutes, stirring frequently.
7. Add the beans and water.
8. Bring to a boil.
9. Reduce the heat to low, cover and simmer for 30 minutes.
10. Uncover and simmer for 30 to 45 minutes, or until the beans are tender. (Add more water if the mixture becomes too dry during cooking.)
11. Stir in the tomato paste and salt.
12. Cook for 2 minutes.
13. Just before serving, stir in the cilantro.

25. BROCCOLI-PEANUT SALAD

INGREDIENTS

- ¼ c white wine vinegar
- 3 Tbsp. canola oil
- 3 Tbsp. peanut butter
- 1 Tbsp. reduced-sodium soy sauce
- ½ tsp salt
- 1 lb. broccoli, tops cut into small florets and stems peeled and chopped
- ¼ c dried cherries, cranberries, or raisins
- ¼ c roasted peanuts, chopped

METHOD

1. Whisk together vinegar, oil, peanut butter, soy sauce, and salt in a large bowl.
2. Toss with broccoli and dried fruit and season with salt to taste.
3. Serve topped with peanuts.
4. Can be made up to 2 days ahead.

36. COCONUT CURRY LENTIL SOUP

INGREDIENTS

- 1 tbsp. coconut oil (or olive oil)
- 1 large onion, chopped
- 2 cloves garlic, minced
- 1 tbsp. fresh ginger, minced
- 2 tbsp. tomato paste (or ketchup)
- 2 tbsp. curry powder
- ½ tsp hot red pepper flakes
- 4 cups vegetable broth
- 1 (400m) can coconut milk
- 1 (400g) can diced tomatoes
- 1.5 cups dry red lentils
- 2-3 handfuls of chopped kale or spinach
- Salt and pepper, to taste
- Garnish: chopped cilantro (fresh coriander) and/or vegan sour cream

METHOD

1. In a stockpot, heat the coconut oil over medium heat and stir-fry the onion, garlic and ginger until the onion is translucent, a couple minutes.
2. Add the tomato paste (or ketchup), curry powder, and red pepper flakes and cook for another minute.
3. Add the vegetable broth, coconut milk, diced tomatoes and lentils.
4. Cover and bring to a boil, then simmer on low heat for 20-30 minutes, until the lentils are very tender.

5. Season with salt and pepper.
6. {Make-Ahead: May be cooled, frozen in air-tight containers, and re-heated over medium-low heat.}
7. Before serving, stir in the kale/spinach and garnish with cilantro and/or vegan sour cream.

27. Roasted Edamame

Ingredients

- 1/4 cup edamame
- 1/4 teaspoon cayenne pepper
- 1/4 teaspoon paprika
- 1 teaspoon olive oil

Method

1. Mix the ingredients in individual bowls.
2. Spread out on a tinfoil lined baking sheet.
3. Roast in a 350 degree oven for 20 minutes, or until crispy.

28. CASHEW BUTTER CAULIFLOWER

INGREDIENTS

- 1 Tbs. Cashew Butter
- 50g Cooked Beetroot
- 150g Cauliflower

METHOD

1. Steam/bake your cauliflower.
2. Using a hand blender or potato masher, pulp the beetroot until smooth.
3. Mix the blended beetroot and cashew butter together until evenly smooth.
4. Once cauliflower is cooked cover it with the beetroot cashew paste.

29. PALAK PANEER WITH TOFU AND SPINACH

INGREDIENTS

INDIAN SPICE RUB

- ½ tsp ground cumin
- 1 tsp ground coriander
- ½ tsp ground ginger
- ¼ tsp ground turmeric
- ¼ tsp ground cinnamon
- 1 tablespoon brown sugar
- 1 package 14-ounce of extra firm organic tofu
- 1 teaspoon extra-virgin olive oil

SPINACH GRAVY

- ⅓ Cup of vegetable broth for sautéing plus ½ cup for spinach gravy
- ⅓ Cup chopped shallots
- 3 garlic cloves, chopped
- 1 tbsp. of grated ginger (grating brings out more flavor than chopping)
- 1 serrano Chile, chopped
- 1 tsp ground cumin
- ⅛ Tsp nutmeg
- Pinch of cayenne

- 1 tbsp. maple syrup
- ¼ cup coconut milk
- Juice of one lime
- ¼ tsp salt or more
- Fresh ground black pepper
- 1 large bunch of spinach (approximately 5 ounces)

METHOD

1. Press the water out of the tofu by wrapping it in a clean dishcloth. Manually press the water out into the dishcloth gently for one minute.
2. Cut into cubes and place in a medium bowl.
3. Make the rub. Combine the cumin, coriander, ginger, turmeric, cinnamon and brown sugar.
4. Sprinkle over the tofu covering evenly.
5. Set aside.
6. Heat ⅓ cup of vegetable broth in a large sauté pan.
7. Season with a pinch of salt and ground black pepper.
8. Add the shallots and sauté for about 3 minutes.
9. Add the ginger, garlic, chili, cumin, nutmeg and cayenne.
10. Sauté until everything is soft and translucent. This should take another 3 minutes.
11. Top the sauté mixture with the spinach.
12. Add ½ cup of vegetable broth. Cover and let steam for 3-4 minutes or until the spinach is wilted,
13. Add the spinach mixture, salt, pepper, maple syrup, coconut milk and lime juice to a food processor and process until smooth.
14. Taste and adjust seasonings.
15. Set aside.
16. Take the same sauté pan, rinse it out, dry with a paper towel and heat the teaspoon of oil.
17. Add the tofu cubes and sauté until they are crisp and brown on all sides. This will take about 3-5 minutes.

18. Remove from sauté pan and set aside.
19. Pour the spinach mixture back into the sauté pan and cook until bubbly about 3-5 minutes.
20. Remove from stove and add in the crispy tofu.
21. Serve with rice and lime wedges and a sprinkle of red chili flakes if you desire.

30. VEGAN MEATBALLS

INGREDIENTS

- ½ cup uncooked lentils
- ⅓ cup vegetable broth
- ½ onion, chopped
- 3 cloves garlic, chopped
- 2 tsp of Italian seasonings
- 2 tbsp. of ground flax
- 4 tbsp. of water
- ½ cup walnuts
- 2 cups of chopped Cremini mushrooms (small pieces)
- ½ cup gluten-free bread crumbs (or regular)
- 1 tsp salt (or more to taste)
- ½ tsp of ground black pepper (or more to taste)
- ¼ cup fresh chopped parsley

METHOD

1. Rinse your lentils with fresh water before boiling to remove any dust and put into a large saucepan.
2. Add 2 cups of water to the saucepan. Be sure to use a large enough saucepan as the lentils will double in size.
3. Bring to a boil, cover, reduce heat and simmer until they are tender. The cooking time is typically 20-25 minutes. Keep a close eye on them just in case you need to add more liquid.
4. When they are done, give them a mash with the potato masher leaving some whole and some mashed.
5. Set aside.

6. Make the flax eggs by combining the 2 tablespoons or ground flax with 4 tablespoons of water.
7. Place in refrigerator to thicken. This usually takes about 10 minutes but you can leave it in longer.
8. Meanwhile, heat a large non-stick sauté pan.
9. Add the walnuts and toast for one minute or two. Make sure you watch them and keep stirring them around so they don't burn.
10. Put the walnuts in a food processor and process until they are medium fine crumble.
11. In the same non-stick saucepan, heat the ⅓ cup of vegetable broth.
12. Season it with the salt and pepper.
13. Add the onion and mushrooms and cook until soft and translucent.
14. Add more vegetable broth if sticking.
15. Add the garlic and cook another minute until soft.
16. Stir in the Italian seasonings.
17. In a large bowl add the cooled, cooked lentils, flax eggs, cooled onion mushroom mixture, bread crumbs, fresh parsley and ground walnuts.
18. Combine well.
19. Taste for seasonings adding more salt, ground black pepper or Italian seasonings,
20. Pre-heat oven to 350 degrees F.
21. Line a baking sheet with parchment paper.
22. Shape the lentil mixture into bowls and pack them tightly so they hold together.
23. Add more bread crumbs if they are falling apart.
24. Place them on the baking sheet about an inch or two apart.
25. Bake for approximately 30 minutes, flipping them over carefully half way through.
26. Serve them with tomato sauce over pasta or make a meatball sandwich.

31. WALNUT POWER SALAD

INGREDIENTS

2 tbsp. coconut butter

½ large yellow onion, thinly sliced

2 cups seedless red grapes, washed and cut in half

2 cups edamame (I did a quick steam-in-the-bag variety)

1 cup uncooked bulgur or other grain

¾ cup walnuts

¼ cup honey

¼ cup water

Fresh baby spinach

Crumbled tofu spicy cheese

Salt to taste

METHOD

1. Melt the coconut butter in a medium saucepan over low heat.
2. Add onions and sauté on low for about 30 minutes, stirring occasionally, until onions are soft, golden brown and almost sweet tasting.

3. While onions are still cooking, pour bulgur and 2 cups water into a saucepan;
4. Bring to a boil and cook for 15 minutes, until most of the moisture has absorbed and the grains are soft enough to eat.
5. Let cool for 15 minutes.
6. When onions are done, stir into the bulgur so the coconut butter is absorbed by the grains.
7. Season with salt.
8. Combine grapes and edamame in a large mixing bowl.
9. Add cooled bulgur and walnuts.
10. Whisk water and honey; pour over mixture and stir well.
11. Add fresh baby spinach and crumbled tofu just before serving.

32. ROASTED MUSHROOM

INGREDIENTS

- 12 oz. cremini (Baby Bella) mushrooms, quartered
- 1 tbsp. + 2 tsp olive oil
- 2 garlic cloves, minced
- ½ tsp crushed rosemary
- ⅛ tsp salt
- ⅛ tsp ground pepper
- 2½ cups shredded romaine lettuce
- ¼ cup pecans, chopped and toasted

THE DRESSING:
- 1½ tbsp.. balsamic vinegar
- ½ tsp Dijon mustard
- ½ tsp agave nectar or honey
- ¼ tsp crushed dried rosemary
- Pinch of salt and pepper
- 1 tbsp. extra-virgin olive oil

METHOD

THE SALAD:
1. Preheat oven to 450 degrees F.
2. Line a baking sheet with parchment paper.
3. In a medium bowl, toss the mushrooms with the olive oil until coated.
4. Add the garlic, rosemary, salt and pepper and toss coat.
5. Spread the mushrooms evenly on the prepared baking sheet.

6. Bake until the mushrooms are brown on the bottom side, about 15 minutes.
7. Turn the mushrooms and bake for an additional 5 minutes.
8. Place the romaine lettuce in a large bowl and combine with the roasted mushrooms, toasted pecans and dressing.
9. Toss to coat and divide between 2 plates. Serve.

THE DRESSING:

1. In a small bowl, whisk together the balsamic vinegar, mustard, agave (or honey), rosemary, salt and pepper. Slowly whisk in the olive oil until combined.

33. VEGAN FRITTATA

INGREDIENTS

- 1¾ cup cooked brown rice
- 1 egg-replacer (you can use flax or Orgran egg replacer)
- 1 yellow pepper, chopped
- 1/2 an onion, chopped
- 4 spring onions/scallions, chopped with the white and green parts separate
- 4 cloves garlic, crushed and chopped
- 3 mushrooms, chopped
- 100g chopped kale
- 100g baby spinach
- Large handful fresh basil leaves
- 1 package firm tofu
- 2 tsp Dijon mustard
- ½ tsp turmeric
- 2 tbsp. soy sauce (or tamari if gluten-free)
- 3 tbsp. nutritional yeast
- 2/3 cup soy or almond milk
- 2 tsp arrowroot
- 1 t tbsp. olive or vegetable oil

METHOD

1. For the crust, pre-heat your oven to 375/190/gas mark 5 and lightly grease your spring form pan.
2. Mix the egg replacer with the cooked rice and then press the rice into the bottom of the pan.

3. Brush the top with a little oil and place in the oven and cook for 10 minutes.
4. Take out and leave to the side.
5. Turn the oven down to 350/180/gas mark 4.
6. Now heat some oil in a frying pan and cook the onion, white part of the scallions and the garlic until they are soft.
7. Add in the pepper and mushrooms and sauté for about 10 minutes.
8. After this, add in the spinach, kale, basil and green parts of the scallions.
9. You may have to do this a little at a time as they will have to wilt down a bit to fit in the pan.
10. As they wilt, turn the heat down to its lowest setting and start with the tofu mixture.
11. For this you will add to a food processor or blender the tofu, mustard, turmeric, soy sauce, nutritional yeast, milk, arrowroot and oil. Blend until you have a smooth consistency.
12. Put the tofu mixture into the greens and stir until everything is combined.
13. Now pour this into the brown rice crust and bake in the pre-heated oven for 40 -50 minutes, depending on how deep or shallow your dish is.
14. Just check it after 35 minutes to make sure it's not too brown.
15. Leave it sitting for about an hour before taking off the sides of the pan.
16. Once you do, allow it to cool before slicing as this will make it set further

34. NOODLE SOUP

INGREDIENTS

- 1/2 block of firm tofu, pressed and drained and cut into cubes
- Corn flour for rolling tofu in
- 2 servings of your favorite rice noodle
- 6 fresh shiitake mushrooms, quartered
- 4 spring onions (scallions), chopped
- 1 red chili, de-seeded and finely chopped
- 3 cloves garlic, crushed and chopped
- A large piece of fresh ginger, peeled and diced finely
- 1 large bunch choi sum (or your favourite green) chopped finely
- Soy sauce or tamari
- 1 tsp chili oil
- 1 tsp toasted sesame oil
- Extra chili, onions, chopped peanuts, fresh coriander and black sesame seeds for garnish

METHOD

1. Pour out some corn flour onto a plate and gently toss the tofu cubes through it so they are coated well.
2. Set aside.
3. Fill a medium – large pot with around 8 cups of water and set over high heat. To this add in your spring onions, chili, garlic and ginger and when it comes to the boil, turn the heat down so it is just simmering.
4. Now add the mushrooms.

5. Whilst those flavors are mixing, heat some oil in a frying pan and throw in the tofu cubes. Fry them until they are golden brown on all sides, adding in a dash of soy sauce right at the end.
6. Put to one side.
7. Now add your noodles to the soup, stir for a minute and then add the chopped choi sum, chili oil, sesame oil and a little soy sauce.
8. Cook until the noodles are soft.
9. Distribute noodles between two bowls and pour soup over each.
10. Top with tofu, extra chili, onions, fresh coriander, chopped peanuts, black sesame seeds and extra chili oil if you wish.

35. VEGGIE BURGER

INGREDIENTS

- Protein Powerhouse Burgers
- 2 15-ounce cans black beans, rinsed and drained
- 1 cup beluga lentils, picked through and rinsed
- 1 cup cooked quinoa
- ½ cup oats, processed into flour (gluten-free if desired)
- ½ cup warm water mixed with 3 tablespoons ground flax
- 2-3 cloves of garlic
- ½ of a red onion, chopped
- 1 red pepper, finely chopped
- 1 tbsp. ground cumin
- ½ tsp cayenne
- 1 tsp Sriracha (or other hot sauce)
- 1 tsp kosher salt
- ¼ tsp freshly ground black pepper
- ½ cup walnuts, chopped
- Roasted Red Pepper Crema*
- 10 ounce jar roasted red peppers, drained
- ½ cup Greek yogurt
- ¼ cup sour cream
- ¼ tsp cayenne
- ½ tsp kosher salt
- 1 tbsp. olive oil

METHOD

1. Preheat the oven to 375.
2. Bring 4 cups of water to a boil. Do not add any salt.

3. Add the beluga lentils to the boiling water, let cook for 5 minutes, and then simmer for 10-15 minutes.
4. When the lentils are tender, drain the excess water and rinse the lentils until the water runs clear.
5. Set aside.
6. Combine the ground flax with the warm water and let sit for 10 minutes.
7. Puree the lentils with 1 can of the black beans.
8. Pour into a large bowl with the remaining black beans, quinoa, oat flour, garlic, red onion, red pepper, walnuts, flax egg, and spices.
9. Taste the mixture and adjust the spices to your liking.
10. Refrigerate the mixture for 1 hour. This isn't necessary, but will make your life a lot easier as you form the patties.
11. To form the patties, grab a handful of the patty mixture and form it into a ball. It will be a bit sticky, but don't fret.
12. Drop onto a parchment-lined sheet, and press down lightly with your fingers to flatten.
13. Repeat with remaining mixture, to form a total of 11 patties.
14. Bake for 12 minutes on one side, flip carefully with a spatula, and bake on the other side for another 12 minutes.
15. Optional - pan fry each patty in a bit of oil to crisping the outside of the burger.
16. While the patties are baking, combine the red peppers, sour cream, Greek yogurt, salt, and cayenne in a food processor.
17. Pulse until smooth, then pour in the oil with the processor running.
18. Set aside until the burgers are ready

36. CHICKPEA CACCIATORE

INGREDIENTS

- 3 cloves garlic, minced
- 1 white onion, diced
- 2 carrots, peeled and diced
- 1 red bell pepper, diced
- ½ tsp dried parsley
- ½ tsp dried thyme
- ½ tsp dried rosemary
- 1 tsp dried oregano
- 1 tsp dried basil
- 1 28 oz. can diced tomatoes
- 1 5.5 oz. can tomato paste
- 1 tbsp. soy sauce
- 1 tbsp. balsamic vinegar
- 2 tsp maple syrup
- 2.5 cups cooked chickpeas (garbanzo beans)
- Salt and pepper, to taste

METHOD

1. Heat a large, non-stick skillet over medium heat.
2. Add the garlic, onion and carrot and sauté in a splash of vegetable broth or water. You can use 1-2 tsp of olive oil for sautéing if you prefer.
3. Cook for 3-4 minutes until the onion starts to soften.
4. Add the red bell pepper and cook another minute or two.
5. Add all the spices, the vinegar, soy sauce and maple syrup and stir to combine.

6. Add the tomato sauce and paste and let simmer lightly for about 15 minutes until it starts to reduce and thicken.
7. Stir in the chickpeas and simmer for another 10-15 minutes until everything is cooked through and the sauce is quite thick.
8. Season with salt and pepper to taste then serve!

37. VEGAN SALAD

INGREDIENTS

- 2-4 cups chopped romaine lettuce or leafy green of choice
- 1 serving red quinoa cooked and chilled (1/4 cup dry)
- ½ cup black beans
- ½ cup corn
- ½ cup jicama, sliced
- ½ cup red pepper, chopped
- 1 small tomato, chopped
- 2 Tbsp. red onion, diced
- Avocado slices and/or pumpkin seeds

METHOD

Mix all ingredients in a salad bowl and garnish with avocado.

38. LENTIL MUNG BEAN LINGUINE SALAD

INGREDIENTS

- 1 package (7.05oz) of organic mung bean linguine
- 1 can organic lentils
- 2 medium leeks, white and light green parts only, cleaned and chopped
- 1 12oz can or jar of artichoke hearts, rinsed and sliced
- Juice of 1 lemon
- ½ yellow onion, diced
- 1 garlic clove, diced
- ½ cup vegan nutritional yeast
- Salt and pepper to taste
- 1 Tbsp. coconut butter

METHOD

1. Melt coconut butter in a pot on the stove over medium-low heat.
2. Add the garlic, onion, and leeks, and cook until caramelized, about 5 minutes.
3. Add the artichokes and sauté for about 3 minutes, and then add the lentils, lemon, salt and pepper.
4. Cover, reduce heat to low, and let simmer for 5-10 minutes.
5. Cook the mung bean linguine al dente per the package instructions and reserve ½ cup pasta water.
6. Transfer the cooked mung bean linguine into the pot with the artichoke, lentil mixture, add the nutritional

yeast and reserved pasta water as needed, and mix all together, adding fresh lemon juice to taste.

39. BLACK BEAN LENTIL SALAD

INGREDIENTS

- 1 cup dry lentils (green or brown)
- 15 oz. can black beans, rinsed and drained
- 1 red bell pepper
- 1/2 small red onion
- 1-2 tomatoes
- Large bunch cilantro stems removed
- Optional: green onion

FOR THE DRESSING
- Juice of 1 lime
- 2 Tbsp. olive oil
- 1 tsp. Dijon mustard
- 1-2 cloves garlic, minced
- 1 tsp. cumin
- 1/2 tsp. oregano
- 1/8 tsp. salt
- Optional: chipotle powder, chili powder, pepper, hot sauce, other seasonings, etc.

METHOD

1. Cook lentils according to package directions, leaving firm not mushy.
2. Drain.
3. While lentils are cooking, make the dressing: place all ingredients in a small bowl and whisk to combine.

4. Set aside.
5. Finely dice the bell pepper, onion, and tomatoes.
6. Roughly chop the cilantro.
7. In a large bowl, place the black beans, bell pepper, onion, tomatoes, and lentils.
8. Add the dressing and toss to combine.
9. Add cilantro, and lightly toss.
10. Serve immediately or chill covered in the fridge for at least an hour to let the flavors combine.

40. GREEK SALAD

INGREDIENTS

- 1/2 cup Cherry tomatoes
- 2 Cucumbers, large
- 1/4 tsp Garlic powder
- 1 Lemon, juice of
- Condiments
- 1/2 cup Kalamata olives
- Baking & Spices
- 1/4 tsp Greek or Italian seasoning
- 1 Pepper
- 4 Pepperoncini peppers
- 1 Salt
- Oils & Vinegars
- 3 tbsp. Olive oil, extra virgin
- 4 oz. spicy tofu cheese

METHOD

1. Mix all ingredients

41. CARROT CAKE OVERNIGHT DESSERT OATS

INGREDIENTS

- 48g (½ cup) Old Fashioned Rolled Oats
- ¾ tsp Ground Cinnamon
- ⅛ tsp Ground Ginger
- ⅛ tsp Ground Nutmeg
- 3 packets Natural Sweetener (stevia, Truvia, etc.)
- pinch Salt
- ¾ cup Unsweetened Vanilla Almond Milk
- ½ tsp Vanilla Extract
- ½ cup Grated Carrots
- 1 tbsp. Chopped Walnuts, Pecans, or Nut Butter of choice

Method

1. In a bowl, stir together the oats, cinnamon, ginger, nutmeg, sweetener and salt.
2. Stir in the milk, vanilla and grated carrots.
3. Cover and refrigerate overnight.
4. Enjoy in the morning.
5. Sprinkle on any of the topping options.

42. BANANA BUCKWHEAT PANCAKES

INGREDIENTS

- 60g (½ cup) Buckwheat Flour
- 1 tsp Double Acting Baking Powder
- ½ tsp Ground Cinnamon
- 2 packets Natural Sweetener (stevia, Truvia, etc.)
- ⅛ tsp Salt
- ½ cup Unsweetened Vanilla Almond Milk
- ½ cup Mashed Ripe Banana
- Optional: ½ tsp Vanilla Extract
- Optional: 2 tbsp. Crumbled Walnuts
- Optional: 1 tbsp. Mini Dark Chocolate Chips

METHOD

1. Spray a flat, nonstick pan with cooking spray and place over medium heat.
2. In a small bowl, whisk together the buckwheat flour, baking powder, cinnamon, sweetener and salt.
3. Stir in the almond milk and mashed banana.
4. Stir in the optional vanilla, walnuts and/or mini chocolate chips, if using.
5. Scoop a large spoonful of batter onto the pan.
6. Cook until the edges look dry and bubbles no longer pop on the surface.
7. Flip and cook for an additional minute or so.
8. Repeat until all the batter is used up.
9. Serve and enjoy!

43. VEGAN COOKIE DOUGH DIP

INGREDIENTS

- 1 15 oz. can of chickpeas, drained and rinsed
- 1/4 cup sunflower seed butter
- 3 tbsp. maple syrup
- 2 tbsp. ground flaxseed (or ground oats/oat flour)
- 1/2 tbsp. vanilla extract
- 1 tbsp. soy milk (or more as needed)
- pinch of salt
- 1/4 cup carob chips or dairy-free chocolate chips

METHOD

1. Combine all ingredients (except the chocolate chips) in a food processor or high speed blender and blend/pulse until well combined and the mixture turns into cookie dough like consistency.
2. Add 1-2 tablespoons of milk as needed.
3. Transfer to a small bowl and fold in the carob or chocolate chips.

44. MAPLE ROASTED PEANUTS RECIPE

INGREDIENTS

- 1 cup maple syrup (Grade B)
- ½ teaspoon salt
- 3 cups peanuts, dry roasted, unsalted
- 1 tsp cinnamon
- 1 tsp vanilla extract

METHOD

1. Cover a baking sheet with parchment or wax paper.
2. In a medium saucepan, whisk together the maple syrup and salt.
3. Fill a large bowl, that's bigger than your saucepan, with cold water. This bowl of water serves two purposes: if you get burned by hot syrup you can dip your hand in it. It will also be used to cool the hot saucepan after the mixture reaches 245F (118C).
4. Bring the mixture to a boil on high heat, covered.
5. Remove cover and reduce heat to medium low so the mixture simmers without boiling over.
6. Do not stir the mixture from now on because natural convection currents will do the stirring for you.
7. Caramelize the maple syrup
8. Insert a candy thermometer and bring the mixture up to 245F (118C).

9. After the mixture reaches this temperature it will start to burn rapidly so 245F (188C) is about the maximum temperature we can caramelize pure maple syrup.

10. Remove from heat and dip the saucepan into the ice water for about 10 seconds to stop the caramelization process.

11. Stir the peanuts and spices into the maple syrup, pour and allow to cool

12. Stir in the peanuts, cinnamon and vanilla extract with a wooden spoon until well incorporated.

13. Pour the mixture onto the baking sheet and separate the nuts as much as possible with two forks.

14. Allow the mixture to cool for about 8 hours before breaking the mixture into individual nut size pieces.

45. CANDIED ALMONDS

INGREDIENTS

- 3 tbsp. s brown sugar
- 2 tbsp. cherry jam
- 2 tsp olive oil
- ½ tsp salt
- 1 cup almonds, raw and unsalted
- ½ tsp almond extract

METHOD

1. Make sugar syrup over heat.
2. In a medium skillet, stir together the brown sugar, cherry jam, olive oil and salt over medium heat until the sugar melts and the syrup bubbles.
3. This should take about 3 minutes.
4. Add the almonds.
5. Stir the almonds and the almond extract until they're evenly coated and toasted.
6. This should take about 5 minutes.
7. Allow the almonds to cool and harden.
8. Spread the nuts out on a piece of parchment paper and separate using two forks.
9. Allow the nuts to cool completely.
10. Nuts can be stored in an airtight container for up to one month.

46. Vegan Chocolate Cake

Ingredients

- 1 ¼ cup all-purpose flour
- 1 cup sugar
- ⅓ cup cocoa powder
- 1 tsp baking soda
- ½ tsp salt
- 1 cup warm water (you may substitute this for coffee)
- 1 tsp vanilla extract
- ⅓ cup vegetable oil
- 1 tsp white or apple cider vinegar
- For the glaze
- ½ cup sugar
- 4 tbsp. margarine or vegan butter substitute
- 2 tbsp. soy milk
- 2 tbsp. cocoa powder
- 2 tsp vanilla extract

Method

1. Prepare the Cake: preheat oven to 350F (177C).
2. In an 8 x 8 inch square pan, mix the flour, sugar, cocoa powder, baking soda and salt with a fork.
3. Add the water or coffee, vanilla extract, vegetable oil and vinegar.
4. Mix the ingredients together.
5. Bake for 30 minutes.
6. Cool on a cooling rack.

7. Prepare the Glaze: in a small saucepan bring the sugar, margarine, soy milk and cocoa powder to a boil, stirring frequently.
8. Simmer for 2 minutes, remove from heat and stir an additional 5 minutes.
9. Stir in the vanilla extract.
10. Glaze the Cake: pour the glaze onto cake and let it cool for one hour.

47. SWEET POTATO QUINOA BOWLS

INGREDIENTS

- 1 cup uncooked quinoa
- 2 small sweet potatoes
- 1 (15 ounce) can black beans, drained and rinsed
- 1/4 cup hemp seeds
- 2 tbsp. sunflower oil (or other high heat oil)
- 2 cups spinach leaves, sliced
- Avocado for topping
- Cilantro-Lime Dressing
- 1 cup cilantro, finely chopped
- 3 tbsp. olive oil
- juice of 2 limes
- 1/4 tsp salt
- 1/2 tsp cumin
- 1 tsp green pepper sauce (or hot sauce)

METHOD

1. Start by preheating the oven to 400°F.
2. Wash and then cut off any gnarly spots on the sweet potato before dicing into 1 inch cubes.
3. Toss with sunflower oil (or any high heat oil) in a baking dish then roast in the oven for 25 minutes.
4. While the potatoes are roasting, cook your quinoa by bringing 2 cups water to a boil over medium heat and add the quinoa to it.

5. Once it is boiling, reduce heat to low and cover with a lid.
6. Cook for 15 to 20
7. While the quinoa is cooking, prepare the dressing by adding all ingredients to a food processor or a small bowl (if you want to chop the cilantro by hand) and mix together.
8. Once potatoes are done, add the hemp seeds to the dish and stir until the potatoes are evenly coated with the seeds.
9. Add the black beans to the dish as well and place back in the oven for 10 minutes.
10. Remove from the oven and set aside.
11. Scoop 1/4 of the quinoa mixture into four separate bowls and then top with (spinach if using) and then the roasted sweet potatoes and beans.
12. Pour 1/4 of the dressing onto each and serve with avocado.

48. CHOCOLATE BANANA HIGH-PROTEIN 'ICE CREAM'

INGREDIENTS

- 2 frozen bananas
- 1 scoop Genuine Health Natural Chocolate Fermented Vegan Proteins +
- 1 Tbsp. cocoa powder
- 1/4 c. coconut milk

METHOD

1. Blend all of the ingredients together in a good blender or a mini food processor until smooth.
2. Serve immediately.
3. You can put the 'ice cream' into piping bag fitted with a larger tip and pipe it into serving dishes.

49. Chocolate Fudge Zucchini Brownies

Ingredients

- 1/2 cup shredded zucchini (100g)
- 1/3 cup applesauce (80g)
- 1 cup plus 2 tbsp. water (270g)
- 2 tsp pure vanilla extract
- 3 tbsp. flax meal (18g)
- 1/2 cup plus 2 tbsp. vegetable or coconut oil (115g)
- 3/4 cup cocoa powder (65g)
- 1 cup coconut flour (135g)
- 1/2 tsp salt
- 1/2 tsp baking soda
- 3/4 cup xylitol or sugar of choice (150g)
- 1/16 tsp pure stevia extract, or 2 extra tbsp. sugar
- 1/2 cup mini chocolate chips, optional

Method

1. Preheat oven to 350F, and line a 9×13 baking dish with parchment paper.
2. Set aside.
3. In a large mixing bowl, whisk together the first 6 ingredients and let sit at least 5 minutes.
4. Combine all other ingredients in a separate bowl, and stir very well.
5. Pour wet into dry, stir until evenly mixed, then pour into the baking dish.

6. Using a full sheet of parchment or wax paper, press down very firmly until the brownie batter evenly covers the pan.
7. Bake 19-20 minutes, and then pat down hard with a pancake spatula or another sheet of parchment.
8. If still undercooked, it's fine. Just fridge overnight and they'll firm up.
9. Let zucchini brownies sit 15 minutes before trying to cut into squares, and if at all possible wait until the next day to eat them.
10. They will be twice as flavorful.
11. As a general rule, cutting brownies with a plastic knife prevents crumbling.

50. Jelly-Filled Muffins

Ingredients

- 1 1/2 cups all-purpose flour
- 3/4 tsp baking powder
- 1/2 tsp baking soda
- 1/2 tsp ground nutmeg
- 1/2 tsp fine salt
- 1 cup plain soy or rice milk
- 1 tsp cider vinegar
- 2 tbsp. cornstarch
- 3/4 cup plus 2 tablespoons granulated sugar
- 1/3 cup vegetable oil
- 2 tsp vanilla extract
- 1/3 cup raspberry, strawberry, or grape jam or preserves
- Powdered sugar, for dusting

Method

1. Heat the oven to 350°F and arrange a rack in the middle.
2. Line a 12-well (1/2 cup) muffin pan with paper liners; set aside.
3. Sift the flour, baking powder, baking soda, nutmeg, and salt into a large bowl.
4. Make a well in the center of the mixture; set aside.
5. In a medium, nonreactive bowl, whisk together the soy or rice milk, vinegar, and cornstarch until the cornstarch has dissolved.
6. Pour this into the well in the flour mixture.

7. Add the granulated sugar, oil, and vanilla and stir with a rubber spatula until combined (there will be a few lumps).
8. Fill each muffin well about three-quarters full.
9. Using a spoon, create a small indentation in the batter by slightly spreading it from the middle out toward the edges.
10. Measure 1 heaping teaspoon of jam or preserves and place the back of the teaspoon inside the indentation.
11. Rotate the spoon, letting the jam slide into the indentation.
12. Repeat in each well.
13. Bake until the tops of the muffins are firm, about 21 to 23 minutes.
14. Set the pan on a wire rack and let cool for 5 minutes.
15. Remove the muffins from the pan and let cool completely on the wire rack.
16. Dust with powdered sugar before serving.

CPSIA information can be obtained
at www.ICGtesting.com
Printed in the USA
LVHW080345160522
718872LV00012B/461

9 781537 164908